How To Drink Tea for Weight Loss

Disclaimer

This book is designed to provide condensed information. It is not intended to reprint all the information that is otherwise available, but instead to complement, amplify and supplement other texts. You are urged to read all the available material, learn as much as possible and tailor the information to your individual needs.

Every effort has been made to make this book as complete and as accurate as possible. However, there may be mistakes, both typographical and in content. Therefore, this text should be used only as a general guide and not as the ultimate source of information. The purpose of this book is to educate.

The author or the publisher shall have neither liability nor responsibility to any person or entity regarding any loss or damage caused, or alleged to have been caused, directly or indirectly, by the information contained in this book.

Table of Contents

How Will This Book Help You?

People have been looking for all kinds of ways to cut their weight down. Some tried all kinds of exercise and diet programs. Others tried consuming various foods and concoctions in the hope of removing extra inches and pounds fast. Others go for extreme measures, even if these entail high cost and the potential of life-threatening side effects. However, only a few people know that what they need to lose weight has always been there for centuries.

This is mainly the objective of this book: "How to Drink Tea for Weight Loss: Healthy Tea Recipes That Will Help You Lose Weight Fast". The main aim of this book is to educate people of the natural wonders of drinking tea and the ways it can help people to lose weight. This book aims to educate people about the unique weight-shaving abilities of tea, as well as its other health-giving properties. It will also show people how to prepare tea the right way so they can lose weight in the most efficient way.

The contents of this book, in no particular order, are as follows.

1. The health properties of tea - Tea is one of the first drinks humans discovered. While it is popular as a drink fit for social gatherings, the main reason for it sticking to the consciousness of communities everywhere is that it helps in improving one's well-being. From how it helps with digestion to how its chemical components stimulate the body to run more efficiently, this book will take a more detailed look on the health properties of tea.

2. The different kinds of tea - Drinking tea in general is always good for you. Of course, not all teas are equal. There are numerous variations of tea available on the market and each of them has different properties. Learning about their different traits would help you appreciate your tea better while improving your knowledge on how tea helps your body.

3. How to prepare tea the right way-True, tea enthusiasts know that the way you prepare tea has a huge say on the quality of the final product. If you do not know how to prepare tea correctly, then you will not get the quality you desire. This book will guide you on how

you can prepare tea like a pro and get a high quality result. Not only will you get great-tasting tea this way, but it will also help in getting the most out of the health-giving benefits of your beverage.

4. How to NOT prepare your tea the right way - Of course, if there is a correct way to prepare tea, there is also an incorrect way to prepare your tea. Of course, these include poor preparation techniques most people do while making their tea. Beyond preparation, this book will also tell you about the ingredients that are not advisable to be added in tea because it either negates the weight-shaving properties of tea or kills the nutritional benefits.

5. Simple healthy tea recipes - There are so many ways to prepare tea, as evidenced by the explosion of numerous tea stores all over the world. This book will teach you how to prepare café-quality tea recipes easily at home. Not only will these recipes put most store-supplied concoctions to shame, but they are also prepared in such a way that it maximizes the health benefits you can get from tea.

Those are just some of the things you can learn from this book. My aim is that by the end of this book, you are able to prepare tea like a boss and lose that excess weight in the process. Get in the best shape of your life with the help of tea!

The Health and Weight Loss Benefits of Tea

"Tea is very healing."

- Kristin Chenoweth

Tea is one of the healthiest drinks you can ever get for yourself. This has been proven often over the years. Our ancestors drank it to keep their body running efficiently. At the same time, modern research has shown that there are scientific facts to match these seemingly lofty claims. From ridding one's body of toxins to shedding off excess pounds, regularly drinking tea greatly helps in keeping you healthy, regardless of your age. This chapter will let you take a look on how regularly drinking tea can improve the state of your health and reduce your weight at the same time.

Numerous health benefits are associated with constant consumption of tea. It does not really matter what kind of tea you prefer consuming. As long as it is of the natural kind (and as long as your drink contains the right ingredients), tea can give a boost to your health in a variety of ways. The following are just some of them.

Detoxification

Removing the toxins from your body is very important. When left unchecked, toxins left inside your body can cause various health problems such as cancers. While other people go to great lengths to rid their bodies of toxins, one of the easiest ways to do it is by drinking tea with regularity. Tea is an amazing source of antioxidants that help in eliminating free radicals. At the same time, tea can stimulate proper bowel movement, which helps in reducing waste materials from digestion.

Prevention of aging

People are looking for all kinds of ways to stave off aging. Drinking tea was clinically proven to protect your body from aging both inside and out. Tea naturally contains antioxidants such as polyphenols that help in eliminating free radicals. By removing free radicals, it is possible to prevent cell destruction. At the same time, studies show that tea helps in strengthening elastin and collagen, 2 proteins naturally found in skin, bones and cartilage. This effect prevents joint erosion and the development of wrinkles.

Stress relief

Relieving stress is one of the keys for holistic health. Tea is one of nature's best stress busters. It is one thing that drinking tea is a welcome treat after a hard day's work. It is another thing that tea is clinically proven to be a cure for stress. A study has shown that the consumption of tea lowers the levels of stress hormones such as cortisol. Also related to this, tea also lowers blood pressure, a common effect associated with stress and is a major stressor in itself. If you feel stressed out, having a cup or two of tea should be a good idea.

Other health benefits

There are other health benefits of tea that has been confirmed by scientific studies or at least currently under serious investigation. Tea is seen to have a positive effect on cardiovascular health as it reduces blood pressure and it is seen to improve the function of the endothelium (the inner layer of blood vessels). At the same time, it might also have a positive effect in reducing a patient's overall risk for developing diabetes. In addition, a study uncovered that it has a protective effect on the retina, which is crucial for maintaining correct eyesight.

Due to the purposes of this book, I have decided to create a completely different topic focused on how tea causes weight loss. It is a fact that drinking tea facilitates weight loss. The surprising fact is that weight loss is accomplished through multiple mechanisms. Each of these ways is beneficial in its own right. Together, these mechanisms make tea such a potent weight-busting drink. Here is the list of the different ways on how tea helps you lose weight.

Tea increases metabolism

Increasing one's metabolic rate is one of the keys to losing weight. The basic rule is that the higher one's metabolism is, the less likely excess calories would be transformed into fat. On the same note, an elevated metabolism causes your body to tap into your fat stores for energy, burning them off on the process. Compounds naturally found in tea such as caffeine and epigallocatechin gallate (EGCG) boost metabolism, helping you burn off food and excess fat at a higher rate. In reality, an increased metabolism helps people lose weight, even without the help of exercise!

Tea helps in mobilizing stored fat

Most people find it difficult to trigger their bodies to use up their excess fat. Drinking tea can significantly help in that regard. Aside from increasing your metabolism, tea also helps in mobilizing fat by triggering changes in your hormonal levels. EGCG inhibits an enzyme that causes the breakdown of epinephrine. By increasing the body's epinephrine levels, body signals to break down fat are emphasized, causing the mobilization of fat bound inside fat cells for metabolic purposes.

Tea helps in increasing fat burn

Have you observed that tea or some components of tea are usually included as an ingredient for weight loss mixes? It has been backed by scientific studies that tea helps in burning fat through a combination of multiple processes. Studies show that those who drink tea burn more fats compared to those who do not. The results become more marked when the person exercises. Briefly, drinking tea combined with exercise will help you achieve significant fat loss.

Tea reduces appetite

As much as calorie burning is a critical part of losing weight, calorie uptake is just as crucial in determining final weight loss. One thing that can significantly help in losing weight is to reduce one's appetite and calorie intake. In numerous studies, it has been observed that calorie intake is reduced in tea drinkers. While further studies must still be done, some studies show evidence that drinking tea may help in appetite regulation. In some animal studies, it is suggested that tea consumption may reduce the amount of fat absorbed from food.

Tea can induce weight loss through multiple ways. One way of evaluating the potency of something is to see how far-reaching its effects are on the subject. If this is the basis, it is safe to assume that tea is one of the best weight loss interventions out there today. Fully natural, highly effective, loaded with positive health effects and with no harmful side effects, it is easy to see why people from all backgrounds are drinking their tea for improved health.

Tea is linked to all kinds of health benefits, with one of the most notable ones in the field of weight loss. By increasing metabolism and potentially inhibiting calorie uptake, it has been proven in numerous studies that tea has a positive effect on weight loss.

Getting to Know the Different Kinds of Tea

"We were in Japan once where they had 30 types of green tea. I thought there was one."

- Billy Corgan

Tea (except those derived from other plants such as peppermint) is usually derived from leaves of the plant Camellia sinensis. While the tea plant is considered native in China, India, and other parts of Asia, it will not be long until the plant will make it around the world. As there are different kinds of tea on the market, it will be interesting to know what the differences between these variants are. Unless specified, all the teas mentioned here are in reality derived from the same tea plant. It is more of the way the leaves are genuinely prepared that creates the different distinctions between these different types of tea.

Without bothering you so much with this introduction, here are some of the most popular kinds of tea you can find in the market today.

White tea

This tea is the purest of all teas. In contrast to the other types, white tea is virtually unprocessed, with the leaves not being subjected to curing or fermentation. To prepare this type of tea, the leaves are simply steamed and then dried. White tea contains only 1-2% caffeine and is distinguished by its light color and flavor. Its mild and delicate taste made it the choice of royalty in Ancient China. As for health benefits, white tea stands out as it is the most potent tea variant for its anticancer properties.

Green tea

This tea is considered as the most popular of them all. This is mainly because of its popularity in Asia. Compared to white tea, green tea leaves are heat-treated to prevent the fermentation of the leaves. Heat treatment is usually done by either roasting or steaming the leaves. After heating, the leaves are rolled and are allowed to dry. Green tea is named as such because they produce a greenish drink once steeped. It has numerous unique health-giving properties. It has the highest EGCG content among all tea variants and is directly linked to preventing diseases such as cancers and hypertension.

Black tea

This tea, while not as popular as its white and green variants, are also being consumed in relatively high amounts around the world. Black tea gained its characteristics through a fermentation process. After fermenting the leaves, they are heated to produce the characteristic black color. This type of tea is mainly characterized by its dark color, strong taste and relatively high caffeine content. Black tea is popular in the medical community because of its caffeine content and its ability to reduce stroke and lung damage risk.

Oolong tea

This type of tea is becoming very popular with the masses these days. Commonly served in Chinese restaurants, this tea is popular for having a full-bodied flavor and distinctive aroma. The preparation of Oolong tea is essentially similar to that of green tea, with some additional steps. After picking the leaves, you need to shake them to induce "bruising", which initiates fermentation and oxidation. The leaves are then roasted or steamed after they have slightly fermented. This form of tea is mainly noted for its ability to lower blood cholesterol levels and potentially stimulate weight loss.

Herbal tea

They are not considered true teas as the leaves used for them are not derived from the tea plant. However, they are fast becoming popular for different reasons. Not only do they bring different flavors into the table, but they can also have unique health-giving properties, depending on the plant where they are derived from. They are usually very versatile to prepare and are becoming widely accepted by the tea-loving community.

More kinds of tea are out there, but these five are the most basic of them all. There are also sub-variants for each type of tea, but that is something you will learn in good time once you are fully into the tea drinking lifestyle. For now, this basic knowledge will serve you well the next time you shop for tea. It will also give you an idea on what to expect once you start drinking and comparing each tea type.

There are different kinds of tea out there. Except for herbal teas, they are all derived from the same tea plant (Camellia sinensis). The way they are prepared mainly sets the differences between each tea type.

How to Make Tea

"I think tea is more zen-like. It requires a different environment."

- Howard Schultz

In many ways, tea is just like its popular counterpart, coffee. Sure, the finished product is much predicated to the quality of the tea leaves themselves, but it also boils down to execution. How one makes his or her tea has a huge say on the quality of the finished product. Do it the right way and you are bound to enjoy a tea of absolutely high quality. Do it wrong and you'll get a drink that is unpleasant tasting and robbed of all its natural goodness. For your benefit, I decided that you must also learn the nuances of preparing tea the right way. A separate chapter will be dedicated to discussing where people go wrong. What this chapter aims to do is to help you learn the basics of preparing the perfect tea.

The water is very important

Water is of central importance in determining the quality of tea. Using the right water enhances the final product in many ways. Go for water that is filtered but not distilled, as distillation makes the water somewhat un-ideal for steeping. You can use tap water, but it is advisable to cool it down for at least 10 seconds before using it for tea.

The vessel is of equal importance

You might be wondering why the most hardcore of tea enthusiasts pay close attention to the utensils. This is because it is very important as well. It is important that the material you use for a tea pot/kettle is non-reactive. Ceramic or glass should be perfect for this purpose. You can preheat the vessel to prevent excess heat loss (more on this later) by adding a little hot water on the vessel where you will steep the tea.

How much tea should I use?

This is an important question most newbies ask when preparing tea. For starters, they usually go for teabags as they are usually proportioned already for a single cup. However, should you go for fresh leaves, the equation becomes a little trickier. It all depends on the type of strength of the tea leaves themselves. To play safe, use one heaped teaspoon of tea leaves per cup. You can master proportions as you become more familiar with your tea. Just remember that not all teas are made equal.

Temperature is critical

On most hot drinks, all you need is to bring the water to a boil, dump the mix, dissolve, and you're good to go. This does not hold true with tea. To get the most out of your tea, you need to steep it at a very specific temperature. For white and green tea, the magic temperature is in between 75 to 85 degrees C, which is just under boiling point. For black and oolong tea, it is at 90 to 100 degrees C, which is at boiling point. As a rule of thumb, fermented tea leaves must be subjected to higher water temperatures. The right temperature ensures efficient steeping and prevents the degradation of compounds.

Steeping

The process of steeping entails the infusion of the contents of tea leaves into the water. Many factors dictate this process. One of them, temperature, was already mentioned earlier. The other important factor for steeping would be time. Different types of tea require different steeping times to infuse all of the contents. As a rule of thumb, the more fermented the leaves are, the longer steeping time it requires. Also, whole leaves require longer steeping than broken leaves. Never steep leaves for too long or else it would result to a bitter blend.

Serving

You can serve your tea either hot or cold. Make sure to remove the leaves before serving to prevent over-steeping and to prevent ingestion of leaves. If you want it hot, we recommend that you serve it immediately after steeping. If you want it cold, you can let it cool down first, place it on the fridge, or add some ice. If you will not consume the tea immediately, you can have it chilled to prevent it from going stale. You can also add some condiments or toppings on your tea to add some flavor in it.

In essence, that is the fundamental steps on how to prepare tea the right way. Get all these right, and you will have superb tea you can drink all day. You will also be able to make the type of tea you will be proud to serve to your friends.

Making tea the right way is essential to get the most out of your drink. It requires attention to detail, but the steps are really very simple. The preparation method is reasonably constant, but the time you will spend in one step depends on the type of tea you're preparing.

How to Not Make Tea

"Brewing a good cup is something not everyone can do, and I loathe bad tea."

- Rod Stewart

If there is a correct way in preparing tea, of course there would be an incorrect way of doing it! These incorrect steps will not just detract the quality of your tea, but it will also hinder its ability to help you lose weight. The degree in which weight loss is compromised is varied, but it is safe to say that to get the most of your tea, you must follow all these steps. Apart from wrong tea preparation, this chapter also contains some tea-drinking habits you must avoid from this point forward.

Beware of diet teas

There used to be a time when there is a so-called diet tea craze. All people must do to lose weight is to drink them and they will instantly start losing weight. However, it is crucial to note that consuming them without moderation can lead to health problems. Many of these teas contain fat blockers, laxatives, and other ingredients that would make you lose weight at the fastest possible way. Potential side effects include nausea, dehydration, diarrhea and even malnutrition.

Avoid tea with added sugar or sweeteners

The reason behind this logic is very simple. Sugar = calories. Extra calories are something you do not want if you are serious about your weight loss goals. If you are in the hunt for teabags (as they are convenient and beginner-friendly), check the label to ensure they are unsweetened. Natural sugar adds extra calories and can make you prone to diabetes. Artificial sugar has some potentially dangerous side effects. If you will be making your own tea, avoid adding sweeteners. You will eventually get used to it.

Not making tea drinking a habit

Some people think that drinking tea would yield instant results. Remember that these drinks are not intended to be a get-thin-quickly formula, and it never was one. To get the most out of tea's health-giving benefits, it would be great to make it a habit. Make an effort to consume at least one glass of tea a day. You can prepare one while making your breakfast. You can even pack a glass of tea as you go outside.

Never use milk for your tea

It has been scientifically proven that adding milk to your tea is counterproductive. While the milk tea craze is sweeping the world, it is actually not the healthiest combination in the world. It has been found that casein, the protein found in milk, creates complexes with the flavonoids found in tea. This renders the flavonoids useless, negating much of the health value of tea. What's more, milk also adds calories you do not need when you are trying to lose excess weight. So yes, avoid the milk tea.

Not combining tea drinking with other healthy habits

Some people wrongly think that as long as they're doing something healthy at the moment, it would compensate all other bad habits they have. This deserves extra emphasis as you try a tea-drinking lifestyle. The benefits you can get from regular tea drinking would be useless if you do not embrace a healthy lifestyle. If you do not have a regular exercise regimen and you continue eating an unbalanced diet filled with excess, you will never get to your ideal weight. Combine regular tea drinking with other health benefits, and you will maximize your weight loss.

You must develop the correct habits when drinking tea. Apart from making tea drinking a habit, what you include in it has a huge say in its ultimate nutritional value. Last, but not least, do not forget that it takes more than just drinking tea to lose weight.

Some Tea Recipes You Can Do At Home

"I take my teabags with me wherever I go."

- Helen Mirren

The rising popularity of tea has resulted to the creation of all kinds of tea recipes. From teahouses to coffee shops and everywhere else in between, it seems like everyone has his or her own version of creating the ideal tea beverage. For the purposes of this book, I have placed the focus on creating tea recipes that would help you accomplish weight loss. While it has been mentioned that drinking tea pure and unadulterated is still the best way to go, getting creative occasionally should help you appreciate tea more. Here are some great tea recipes for weight loss you can prepare at home.

Lemon Ginger Cooler

With your experience with iced tea, you just know that lemon and tea simply works very well together. The addition of ginger in the mix not only gives a new dimension to the flavor of this drink, but it also adds a distinctive flavor too. Complementing the fat-shredding powers of tea is the ability of ginger to trigger weight loss. Ginger root helps in burning fat and reduces the reproduction rate of adipose cells.

Servings: Good for 2

Ingredients: 4 teaspoons White or Black tea, lemon grass, lemon peel, ginger root

Directions: Steep all ingredients in hot water. Ideally, the temperature must be at 195 degrees F. The drink should be ready in 3 to 5 minutes. Serve hot.

Spiced Green Tea Smoothie

Do you want to add some spice to your tea? This recipe can add spice to your drink, literally. The heat coming from the spices is the perfect contrast to the cool presented by the tea and ice. To sweeten the pot, each serving has less than 100 calories and it is loaded with a ton of metabolism boosting goodness. We can bet tea smoothies are not made like this in your local coffee shop.

Servings: Good for 2

Ingredients: ¾ cup prepared green tea, 2 tablespoons lemon juice, ¼ teaspoon cayenne pepper, 1 piece pear (chopped), 2 tablespoons fat-free yogurt, 2 teaspoons agave nectar, ice

Directions: Mix all ingredients inside a blender. Pulse until mixture becomes smooth. Drink while it is cold.

Green Tea Tonic

This is a recipe inspired by a popular Dr. Oz tea recipe called the Tangerine Weight-Orade. This remarkably simple recipe is one of the best slimming tea recipes you can find out there. It combines 2 weight-busting ingredients: green tea and tangerine. This green tea tonic is great for the summer days as it is cool and refreshing. Shredding off extra pounds while chilling out: who wouldn't want that, right?

Servings: Good for 8

Ingredients: 8 cups (2 liters) green tea, 1 tangerine or orange (sliced), 1 handful of mint leaves

Directions: While brewing the tea, mix in the tangerine so it infuses together with the tea. Cool down the mixture for around 5 minutes and then add the mint leaves. Refrigerate overnight before serving.

Green tea elixir

The degree of difficulty in preparing this tea is significantly higher compared to the other drinks included in this list. This drink will demand you to prepare well in advance, but I swear you are going to love the result once it is all complete. Provided you do not add any sugar or sweetener, this drink should help you a lot as you try to lose weight. It's refreshing taste and fat-burning characteristics will keep you coming back for more.

Servings: Good for 8

Ingredients: ¼ cup green tea leaves, ¼ cup lemon juice, 1 cup ginger syrup (more on this later), ¼ cup pomegranate molasses, mint leaves, lemon slices for garnish

Directions (for ginger syrup): Mix ¼ cup water and ½ cup sugar together in a saucepan. Whisk this mixture together as the syrup comes to a boil. Stir in 2 tablespoons of shredded ginger. Cool the mixture down then refrigerate overnight.

Directions (for tea): Heat 2 ½ liters of water up to 170 degrees F. Turn off heat then place tea in water. Let the tea leaves steep in the water for 5 minutes. Strain mixture and discard the leaves. Stir ginger syrup, lemon juice, and pomegranate molasses. Add 6 cups of cold water and stir. Let the mixture chill overnight. Serve over ice and garnish with lemon slices and mint leaves.

Lavender white tea

White tea is highly notable for its smooth taste. Combine this with the equally smooth taste of lavender and you get a drink that is fit for warm summer days. This drink is very simple to prepare and would help you lose weight in no time. To sweeten the pot, getting lavender for your drink is not as hard as you think.

Servings: Good for 4

Ingredients: 4 bags or 4 tablespoons white tea leaves, 2 teaspoons fresh lavender blossoms, sprigs of lavender for garnishing

Directions: Simmer 2 cups of water in a saucepan. Once it boils, turn off the heat and add both tea leaves and lavender. Steep for 5

minutes and then strain the mixture. Let the prepared tea cool down. Pour mixture on glasses filled with ice. Garnish with lavender sprigs if desired.

Green tea cranberry spritzer

This is the type of drink you will be more than comfortable to share with your friends during parties. Compared to other spritzers, this one is completely healthy and can help you lose some pounds to boot! I would bet that your folks would not even recognize that it is a full-fledged "diet drink" and made using fresh green tea! If you want to impress on your next party, then you should definitely add this mix on the menu.

Servings: Good for 4

Ingredients: 4 tablespoons fresh green tea leaves or 4 bags green tea leaves, ½ cup cranberry juice, 2 cups soda water, 1/3 cup sugar (optional)

Directions: Steep tea in 2 cups of hot water for 2 to 5 minutes. Heat 1/3 cup water in a saucepan and let the sugar completely dissolve in it. Mix together tea, sugar mixture, and cranberry juice. Distribute mixture into 4 glasses and then fill them up with soda water.

Green tea, kiwi, and mango smoothie

Everybody loves his or her smoothies. Something that is used to be a staple only at the tropics, it is fast becoming a favorite for people all over the world. This fruity smoothie loaded with green tea can give you all the sweetness you need (without the excess) and more. It has an abundance of vitamins as well as antioxidants and compounds that aid with weight loss and digestive health. If you are aiming to lose weight for health, do it with style by having a glass of this lovely smoothie.

Servings: Good for 4

Ingredients: 2 yellow mangoes (frozen and diced), 3 ripe kiwis (quartered), ¼ cup honey, ¾ cup unsweetened yogurt, ½ cup baby spinach, 2 tablespoons green tea, 2 tablespoons water, 2 cups ice cubes, ½ teaspoon lime rind

Directions: In a blender, place mango, half of the yogurt and honey, lime rind, and water. Process the mixture while stirring it occasionally. Place this mixture on glasses and store them in the freezer. Meanwhile, place the remaining yogurt and honey, kiwi, spinach, green tea, and ice on the blender. Once blended, place this mixture on the glasses filled with the mango mixture. Serve immediately.

Blueberry and tea smoothie

How about this for a detox drink? Blueberries and tea are both extremely rich with antioxidants that keep cells functioning youthfully. What's more, these antioxidants also have a preventive function against diseases such as cancer. This smoothie will not just help you get all the antioxidants you will need, but it would also help in increasing metabolism for weight loss. Furthermore did we mention that it's an extremely yummy drink too?

Servings: Good for 4

Ingredients: 2 cups fresh blueberries (frozen), 2 cups white tea (chilled), 1 cup fat-free yogurt, 2 tablespoons almonds, 2 tablespoons flaxseed, ice

Directions: Mix all ingredients together in a blender and process until smooth.

All kinds of tea recipes are out there and each one can help you achieve weight loss. Those are just some samples. Feel free to create your own mixes, provided you do not include the bad stuff in there. Good luck and have fun!

How to Apply What You've Learned?

Drinking tea is one of the best decisions you will ever make when it comes to your own health. Beyond losing weight, tea drinking as a habit can help in making your body stronger. Losing those excess pounds will be very beneficial for your health in so many ways, but the impact of tea in your health goes beyond that. It protects your cells, keeps your digestive tract running in high gear, and improves your immunity too.

Proper preparation of tea is important so you can get the most out of it. It all starts with the selection of tea. While all kinds of tea are good and of equal value, each has specific requirements, so you can get the best out of them. From water temperature to steeping time, all these factors are critical to make the best tea possible. It may take time to get used to, but trust me, all these are very important.

Apart from proper preparation, it is important to consider what you would add to your drink. While it takes some time to get used to it, I recommend that you drink your tea in its pure form. This maximizes the weight loss potential of tea and keeps calorie consumption at a minimum. If you shall add some toppings, I advise that you stick with healthy ones such as fruit and spice. Some ingredients such as sugar and milk are not recommended as these nullify many of the weight-shaving properties of tea. There are numerous healthy tea recipes out there. Feel free to research and experiment.

Last but definitely not the least, I would recommend that you combine tea drinking with other healthy habits. Get enough exercise. Eat a balanced diet. Take control of your daily habits so that your body would be in the best shape. A little discipline and a well-rounded lifestyle can go a long way in accomplishing your fitness goals.